Core Exercises for Seniors Over 60

A Workout Guide for Better Mobility, Posture & Balance

Oliver Bates

Table of Content

ABOUT THIS BOOK

In this book, we're embarking on an enlightening journey! Every page is packed with useful insights, yet it remains as straightforward as a chat with an old friend. We'll kick things off by unraveling the mysteries of our bodies, zooming in on the core. Then, brace yourself for a deep dive into hands-on core exercises, categorized by their positions. And to wrap things up? A dash of real-world application to bring it all home.

In Chapter 1, we'll dive into the fascinating journey of aging and explore tricks to keep muscle loss at bay. We'll also map out the maze of core muscles and unveil how powering up your core can amp up your daily life. And hey, don't skip our fun core strength quiz – it's your golden ticket to gauge where you stand!

Chapter 2 dives into the exciting journey of building core strength—and guess what? You don't need any fancy equipment! Discover common pitfalls to avoid and snag some top-notch advice to maximize every moment of your workout.

Chapter 3 focuses on seated core exercises. Many are taken aback by the revelation of how secure, gentle, yet profoundly potent such exercises can be for individuals across age groups. A collection of twelve dynamic core exercises is showcased, each effortlessly performed while nestled in a chair.

Chapter 4 dives into the exciting world of standing core exercises, adding a delightful twist to your regular workout regimen. When you train your core muscles while standing, you're introducing a game-changing element that keeps both you and your muscles guessing. The chapter features a dazzling array of twelve standing exercises designed to supercharge your core strength in new and dynamic ways!

Chapter 5 focuses on mat core exercises. Expecting a monotonous list of sit-ups? Prepare to be surprised! We'll unveil twelve top-tier core workouts you can perfect lying down. And here's a hint: you won't find a single sit-up or crunch on the list!

HOW TO USE THIS BOOK

Not just a deep dive into the core and its incredible advantages, this book also serves as a treasure trove of fifty handpicked core-boosting exercises you can kickstart right away! Plus, we've got an extra cherry on top: ten warm-up and cool-down routines to make sure you're getting the most out of your workout. Think of this book as your go-to resource, a well-thumbed manual you'll revisit as you evolve in your journey to fortify that core.

And here's the kicker:

Each exercise spotlighted in this guide comes complete with:

1. Name of the exercise
2. Easy step-by-step instructions
3. A variation of the exercise or a way to level up and make the exercise more challenging.
4. Safety tips and things to watch out for to avoid injury.

Get ready to nail those poses! Every exercise in this book comes with easy-to-follow steps, detailing exactly where your hands, feet, head, and body should be. You won't have to guess—you'll know!

Now, how you use this book is entirely up to you—and tailored to fit your lifestyle, skill level, and objectives. You've got options! For the detail-oriented among us, you could work your way through each exercise and chapter, systematically building your core strength. Want to shake things up? Feel free to mix and match the exercises to create your own daily workout routine. And if you're all about convenience, we've got you covered. Just flip to the end of the book and you'll find pre-planned weekly schedules ready for you to follow.

The bottom line? Pick a method that you can commit to—one that meshes with your life. Your pathway to a more robust core is just a few dedicated workouts away. So roll up those sleeves and let's get started! Your stronger, more stable core is just around the corner, waiting for a bit of your effort to bring it to life!

Aging is a fact of life we can't dodge. However, let's be clear: slipping into weakness and losing muscle isn't a package deal with growing older. The power to age gracefully, full of vigor and stability, lies in understanding our bodies, gaining wisdom about muscle degeneration, and taking conscious, deliberate steps to counteract it. That's what this book aims to help you do.

I wrote this book with one primary goal in mind: to be your loyal companion on this journey toward a healthier, more robust you. Why? So that we can all rock the later chapters of our lives with energy and zest. I hope you find this book to be your go-to guide for fortifying your core and anchoring your stability.

Before you dive into any new exercises or activities, make sure to get the green light from your healthcare provider. Safety first!

Finally, a huge thank you for choosing my book. If you find it valuable, I'd be incredibly grateful if you could take a moment to leave a review on Amazon. Your insights not only help me but also guide others who are on the lookout for a resource like this. To me, that's priceless.

INTRODUCTION

In every stage of life, health is your most valuable asset. However, as we age, our approach to health needs to evolve. The golden years of life present unique challenges but also unprecedented opportunities. The objective of this book, "The Golden Path: Core Exercises for Seniors," is to guide you through these years with a specific focus on strengthening your core muscles. These muscles serve as the cornerstone of your overall fitness, affecting everything from balance to posture, and even influencing your cardiovascular health.

When we talk about the 'core,' we often imagine six-pack abs sported by young athletes or fitness models. But in reality, the core is a complex set of muscles that extends far beyond the abs, including everything from your lower back to your pelvic floor. For seniors, maintaining core strength isn't about aesthetics; it's about quality of life. A strong core helps in keeping you upright, supporting your spine, improving balance, and reducing the risk of falls and injuries—challenges that often accompany aging.

Perhaps you are new to exercise, or maybe you are looking to adapt your existing fitness regimen to better suit your needs as a senior. Either way, this book is designed for you. Each chapter is tailored to provide you with comprehensive information and practical advice, including anatomical explanations, the effects of aging on core strength, and safety measures to consider before embarking on your fitness journey. You'll also find an array of core exercises, from isometric to dynamic, as well as nutritional advice and mental practices to complement your physical training.

Remember, age is just a number, but a strong core is timeless. What activities in our daily routine rely on our core strength? Almost every single one!

- Perching on a seat
- Rising from a lying position or from sitting
- Glancing over your shoulder
- Lifting objects or carrying parcels
- Bending down to fasten your shoelaces.
- Putting on clothes
- Bathing or showering
- Stretching to grab something from a high shelf.
- Cleaning activities such as using a vacuum, broom, or mop.

- Engaging in DIY tasks like nailing, slicing, or using a screwdriver
- Engaging in sports like cycling, swimming, bowling, golf, tennis, rowing, jogging, or simply taking a stroll.

To keep enjoying our daily routines independently, it's crucial that we keep our core muscles in tip-top shape. Imagine needing a helping hand for every little task! Age naturally causes our muscles, especially our core, to lose some of their vigor. This could be due to various reasons, from past injuries to long bouts of inactivity. But don't get disheartened.

Exercise is not just about living longer; it's about living better. You've accumulated years of wisdom and experience; it's time to add physical vitality to your well-earned life attributes. "The Golden Path: Core Exercises for Seniors" is not just a book; it's your companion and guide to a healthier, more fulfilling life.

THE ESSENCE OF CORE

The Essence of Your Core—it's not just a phrase; it's a mantra for a life full of zest and vitality. Your core isn't simply a cluster of muscles residing in your midsection. No, it's the epicenter of your physical well-being, the engine room of your body, the very anchor that holds everything else in alignment.

When you invest in your core, you're not merely doing sit-ups or leg lifts. You're building a fortress for your spine, you're erecting scaffolding for your posture, and you're creating a foundation for every move you make—be it lifting a grandchild high up into the air, mastering the art of gardening, or simply standing up straight without a wince of back pain.

Having a robust core doesn't just empower you physically. It acts as a catalyst for mental well-being. Imagine not being bound by limitations, where your age is merely a chronological number, not a dictation of your physical ability.

In this chapter, we're going to explore the fascinating changes our bodies go through as we age. Then, we'll dive into the nitty-gritty of what muscles actually constitute our core. Curious about the perks of a rock-solid core? We've got that covered too! And to top it off, we've got a quick but revealing quiz to help you gauge just how robust—or not—your core really is.

Our bodies and aging

The core is often described as the "powerhouse" of the body, and rightly so. It is a group of muscles that serves as a fulcrum around which all physical activities revolve. Yet, the significance of core strength tends to be overlooked, especially in the context of senior health and fitness.

When you're younger, a lot of physical abilities are taken for granted. You can easily pick up your grandchildren, bend down to tie your shoes, or carry groceries without a second thought. However, as you age, these seemingly mundane activities can become challenging. This is largely because the core muscles, like other parts of the body, tend to weaken with age.

Aging is an inevitable journey we all embark on. But hey, let's get real: hitting the big 6-0 doesn't mean you've got one foot in the grave. Maybe that was the narrative centuries ago when living past 60 was something of a miracle. Fast forward to today, and people are rockin' their 80s and even 90s with verve and vitality!

Here's another twist: the "senior" label comes with its own sub-genres. Picture this:

Young-Old: Think ages 65 to 74. You're basically the fresh-faced "newbies" of the senior world!

Middle-Old: This is the 75 to 84 crowd. You're the seasoned pros, hitting your stride and enjoying the wisdom that comes with it.

Old-Old: At 85 and beyond, you're the grandmasters, the true connoisseurs of life who've seen it all and lived to tell the tale!

The physical prowess of a 65-year-old can be worlds apart from an 85-year-old, and the difference isn't just a matter of years on a calendar. It's also shaped by an array of factors, from the kind of food on their plate to the quality of sleep they get at night. Add to that the mix of mental sharpness, general fitness, and existing health conditions, and you'll see that age really is just a number when it comes to physical capability.

Let's get real about age—there are two kinds to consider. You've got your chronological age, which ticks along year by year, whether you like it or not. But then there's your biological age, which is a whole different ball game. That's the age your body feels and functions at, and guess what? You have a say in it.

Imagine two people, both 72 years young. One battled breast cancer and emerged on the other side with a zest for life. She feasts on a rainbow of fruits, veggies, and lean proteins, spends her weekends nailing putts on the golf course, incorporates stretching into her daily routine, and winds down with jigsaw puzzles that keep her mind razor-sharp. Contrast that with another 72-year-old who's got some arthritis in his hands, no other major health flags, but a pantry full of processed foods and a love for couch-potato life. He complains of brain fog, rarely exercises, and is a daytime TV binge-watcher.

Both individuals are the same age if you're counting candles on a cake, but take a look under the hood and their bodies are aging at completely different speeds. So when it comes to aging, it's not just about the years in your life, but the life in your years. And that, my friend, is largely up to you.

Your body is like a bustling city, teeming with various kinds of cells that each have their own jobs and lifespans. Just like some buildings are torn down and rebuilt while others stand the test of time, so it is with our cells. Skin cells are the city's scaffolding—constantly being torn down and renewed. On the other end of the spectrum, our brain cells are the historic landmarks—once they're gone, they're irreplaceable. Now, let's talk about muscle cells. They're like self-sustaining, eco-friendly buildings—capable of renewing themselves.

But here's the catch: as we hit the senior years, it's like our city starts to lose some of its infrastructure. Our muscles weaken and shrink, making us more prone to falls and less mobile. The good news? Turning this around is totally doable and doesn't require a complete lifestyle overhaul.

Cue the science: A 2018 study by McCormick and Vasilaki points out the key lifestyle tweaks that can make all the difference in maintaining your muscle mojo. So yes, it's not just about how many birthdays you've celebrated, but how you've geared up for the years ahead.

- Protein Power-Up: Did you know that close to 40% of folks aged 50 and above aren't getting enough protein? Don't be part of the statistic! Protein is your muscle's best friend, so let's ramp up that intake.

- Cardio Kings and Queens: Whether you're walking the dog, jogging in the park, biking on a trail, or doing laps in the pool, you're doing wonders for your heart and muscles. Plus, who doesn't want lungs that can sing all the verses of your favorite song without missing a beat?

- Strength in Resistance: Forget the myth that weights are just for bodybuilders! A little weightlifting, some bodyweight exercises, or even using resistance bands can help your muscles grow and get stronger. You'll be flexing those biceps in no time.

- Flex and Flow: It's not all about pumping iron and pounding pavement. Gentle activities like stretching, yoga, and core exercises can make you limber and strong. Trust us, your muscles will thank you for the balance and flexibility!

Opting to tweak our everyday routines can be a game-changer in combating the decline of muscle power and core stability that comes with aging.

Understanding Your Core

In the journey toward understanding how to strengthen the core, especially for seniors, it is essential first to know what constitutes the core muscles. Far from being just your "abs," the core is a complex group of muscles that serve as a central link connecting your upper and lower body. These muscles are engaged in nearly everything you do, from picking up a pencil to swinging a golf club.

What Constitutes the Core?

When we speak about the core, we generally refer to several groups of muscles:

- Rectus Abdominis: Located along the front of the abdomen, this is the most well-known abdominal muscle and is often referred to as the "six-pack" due to its appearance in physically fit individuals.
- Obliques: These muscles are on the sides of your abdomen and come in two varieties—internal and external. They are responsible for the rotation and lateral movement of the spine.
- Transverse Abdominis: This is the deepest of the abdominal muscles and wraps around your spine for protection and stability.
- Erector Spinae: These muscles run along your neck to your lower back and are essential for standing and lifting objects.
- Multifidus: This is a series of muscles attached to the spinal column, assisting in a variety of subtle movements and playing a key role in spinal stability.
- Hip Flexors: Located in the front of the pelvis and upper thigh, these muscles are essential for lifting the knees and bending at the waist.

- Gluteus Maximus, Medius, and Minimus: These are the muscles of your buttocks and are crucial for hip movement, stability, and power.

- Pelvic Floor: These muscles are like a sling that holds your internal organs in place, including the bladder and bowel in men, and the bladder, bowel, and uterus in women.

How Do These Muscles Work Together?

These muscle groups work cohesively to support the spine, allow twist and bend, maintain upright posture, and help in activities like walking, lifting, and even breathing. When one part of this system is weak, it affects the efficiency and effectiveness of the others, often leading to imbalance and, subsequently, to injury.

Changes with Aging

As we age, our muscle mass decreases, affecting all muscle groups including the core. The loss of muscle mass affects the ability to perform tasks that may have once been simple. For example, lifting groceries, climbing stairs, or even getting up from a sitting position can become increasingly difficult. The weakening of the pelvic floor muscles can also lead to issues like incontinence, which can significantly affect the quality of life for seniors.

The Role of Connective Tissues

In addition to muscles, it's important to consider the role of tendons and ligaments. These connective tissues link muscles to bones and bones to bones, respectively. With age, these tissues lose some of their elasticity, making them more susceptible to injury. Strengthening your core, therefore, also plays a role in maintaining the health of these connective tissues.

The Neurological Aspect

Core strength is not only about muscles and bones; it's also about the nerves that control them. The neuromuscular system is responsible for coordinating your movements and balance. Therefore, a strong core enhances the communication between your nervous system and muscles, allowing for more robust, precise movements, which is particularly beneficial for seniors, for whom fine motor skills might be declining.

Understanding the anatomy and physiology of your core is the first crucial step in knowing how to strengthen it effectively. Armed with this knowledge, you can now appreciate the science behind the exercises and regimes that will be outlined in the coming chapters. This will not only make you more conscious of each movement but also help you in understanding what particular areas you need to focus on to better improve your core strength and, consequently, your overall well-being.

The Risk Factors of a Weak Core

While a strong core is the cornerstone of overall health and physical ability, especially in later years, a weak core comes with its own set of problems. Understanding the risks associated with having a weak core can serve as a motivating factor to take proactive steps to strengthen it.

Increased Risk of Falls

One of the most immediate risks of having a weak core, particularly for seniors, is an increased susceptibility to falls. A strong core contributes to better balance and stability, helping you negotiate uneven terrain and respond to shifts in your center of gravity. Falls are a significant health concern for seniors, often leading to fractures, which can have cascading negative effects on overall health.

Poor Posture

Over time, a weak core can lead to poor posture. Core muscles support the spine and help maintain an upright position. When these muscles are weak, the tendency to slouch or hunch increases, putting additional pressure on the spine and contributing to chronic back pain.

Lower Back Pain

The core muscles work in harmony to stabilize the spine during movement. When the core is weak, other muscle groups, such as those in the back, have to compensate. This often leads to muscle imbalances and, consequently, to lower back pain.

Reduced Functional Mobility

Everyday activities like bending down to pick something up, reaching for items on a high shelf, or even getting in and out of a car can become arduous tasks when your core is weak. Reduced functional mobility limits your ability to live independently, affecting your quality of life.

Reduced Respiratory Function

Though not immediately obvious, a weak core can compromise your respiratory function. Muscles like the diaphragm are a part of the core system and are essential for effective breathing. A weak core can lead to shallow breathing, reducing oxygen supply to the body, affecting stamina and potentially worsening conditions like COPD (Chronic Obstructive Pulmonary Disease).

Musculoskeletal Injuries

With a weak core, you're more susceptible to musculoskeletal injuries. Activities that you once found easy can become hazardous, not only due to reduced strength but also because of reduced stabilizing capability of the core muscles, leading to strains and sprains.

Poor Digestive Health

Core muscles are also linked to your digestive system. A weak core can result in poor posture, which, in turn, can lead to digestive problems like acid reflux and constipation. Though it may sound surprising, strengthening your core can help improve your digestive processes.

Reduced Mental Health

A weak core and the resulting limitations on physical activity can lead to a decline in mental health. Exercise is known to release endorphins, which are natural mood lifters. Limitations in physical activity can lead to feelings of depression, anxiety, and contribute to a general sense of malaise.

Reduced Quality of Life

Collectively, all these factors significantly impact your quality of life. Whether it's enjoying time with grandchildren, traveling, or simply living independently, a weak core can make all these activities challenging and less enjoyable.

Understanding the risks associated with a weak core, particularly for seniors, emphasizes the importance of the core-strengthening activities and practices outlined in this book. In the subsequent chapters, we'll explore how to safely and effectively build core strength, enhancing not only your physical well-being but also your overall quality of life.

Benefit of strengthening your core

Having explored the anatomy of the core and the risks associated with a weak core, particularly in seniors, it's now time to focus on the brighter side of the spectrum: the numerous benefits that come with a strengthened core. While some of these advantages might seem immediately apparent, others are less obvious but equally impactful, especially as we age.

Improved Balance and Stability

A strong core acts as a stabilizing center of power that supports and enables all types of movements. This is particularly crucial for seniors, for whom balance, and stability can become compromised. Core strength reduces the risk of falls, one of the most common causes of injury in older adults.

Enhanced Posture

Core muscles support the spine and affect the way we hold our back, neck, and shoulders. With a strong core, maintaining an upright posture becomes more natural, reducing strain on the spinal column. Good posture not only makes you look taller and more confident but also prevents a multitude of health issues ranging from back pain to nerve compression.

Pain Reduction

A strong core can significantly alleviate lower back pain by providing better spinal support. This can be life-changing for seniors who suffer from chronic back pain, a common ailment that affects quality of life.

More Efficient Movement

Your core is involved in almost every movement your body makes, from swinging a golf club to bending down to tie your shoes. A strong core makes these movements more efficient and less taxing on the body. This improvement can translate into better performance in physical activities and less fatigue in daily life.

Improved Respiratory Function

As previously discussed, core muscles like the diaphragm play a significant role in breathing. Strengthening your core can lead to more efficient respiratory functions, allowing for better oxygenation of the body and improved stamina, crucial for people with respiratory issues or those who simply wish to improve their athletic performance.

Better Digestive Health

While it may not be obvious, a strong core can positively affect digestive processes. Improved posture allows the digestive tract to assume its natural alignment, making the process of moving food through the system more efficient, which can help in reducing issues like constipation and acid reflux.

Enhanced Athletic Performance

For those seniors who engage in sports or regular physical activities, a strong core can lead to improved performance. Whether it's golf, tennis, swimming, or even jogging, a robust core contributes to better balance, more powerful movements, and reduced risk of injury.

Increased Functional Independence

Perhaps one of the most critical benefits, especially for seniors, is the increase in functional independence that comes with a strong core. Tasks such as lifting groceries, climbing stairs, or caring for grandchildren become easier, allowing for a more independent and fulfilling life.

Mental Health Benefits

Physical strength often translates into emotional strength. Regular exercise, including core-strengthening activities, can significantly improve mental health by reducing symptoms of depression and anxiety. The endorphins released during exercise act as natural mood lifters, and the increased physical capabilities can boost self-esteem and overall well-being.

Longer, Healthier Life

In the bigger picture, a strong core contributes to longevity and a higher quality of life. With reduced risks of falls, improved functional abilities, and better health indicators, people with strong cores are better equipped to enjoy their senior years to the fullest.

Understanding these benefits provides a comprehensive view of the significance of core strength at any age, but especially for seniors.

Test Your Core

Curious about the strength of your core muscles? Dive into the quiz below to get a feel for where you stand! Remember, this is a judgment-free zone—just be truthful with your answers. The goal is to discover how your core can become even stronger!

Core Strength Quiz for Seniors

Before diving into core-strengthening exercises, it's beneficial to assess your current core strength and awareness. This quiz is designed to help you understand where you stand and to guide you in choosing the best exercises suitable for your level.

Note: This quiz is not a substitute for professional medical advice. Always consult with a healthcare provider before starting any new exercise regimen.

How To Take the Quiz:

Answer each question honestly. Tally your points to find out your core strength level at the end.

1. How often do you engage in physical exercise that targets the core?

- Never (0 points)
- Rarely, less than once a month (1 point)
- Occasionally, a couple of times a month (2 points)
- Regularly, at least once a week (3 points)

2. Can you maintain a plank position for 30 seconds?

- No (0 points)
- Struggle but can do it (1 point)
- Yes, comfortably (2 points)

3. Do you experience back pain?

- Frequently (0 points)
- Occasionally (1 point)
- Rarely or never (2 points)

4. How would you describe your posture?

- Poor, I slouch often (0 points)
- Fair, I catch myself slouching but correct it (1 point)
- Good, I maintain an upright posture most of the time (2 points)

5. Can you rise from a chair without using your hands for support?

- No (0 points)
- With difficulty (1 point)
- Yes, easily (2 points)

6. How's your balance? Can you stand on one foot for 10 seconds without support?

- No (0 points)
- With difficulty (1 point)
- Yes, easily (2 points)

7. Do you participate in activities that require balance and coordination (like dancing, golf, or even brisk walking)?

- No (0 points)
- Occasionally (1 point)
- Regularly (2 points)

8. Can you climb a flight of stairs without holding onto the railing for support?

- No (0 points)
- Yes, but with difficulty (1 point)
- Yes, easily (2 points)

9. How often do you experience digestive issues like bloating, acid reflux, or constipation?

- Frequently (0 points)
- Occasionally (1 point)
- Rarely or never (2 points)

10. Do you feel fatigue setting in quickly during physical activities?

- Yes, often (0 points)
- Occasionally (1 point)
- Rarely or never (2 points)

Scoring:

0-8 points: Low Core Strength: Your core could benefit significantly from targeted exercises. The following chapters will offer beginner-level exercises tailored for you.

9-16 points: Moderate Core Strength: You have a decent level of core strength but there's room for improvement. The upcoming chapters will provide intermediate exercises to boost your core strength.

17-20 points: High Core Strength: Excellent! Your core is strong. You can focus on maintenance and perhaps challenge yourself with more advanced exercises detailed in later chapters.

Armed with the knowledge of your current core strength level, you can now proceed to the following chapters that offer a range of exercises and activities designed to build your core strength efficiently and safely.

DEVELOPING A STRONG CORE

You've taken the quiz, so you have an idea where your core strength stands. Now it's time to get into the nuts and bolts of developing a strong and resilient core. The upcoming guidance aims to help you progress safely and effectively, irrespective of your current fitness level. Before we delve into the specific exercises, let's outline some foundational principles that will guide your core-strengthening journey.

Understand The Importance of Progression

Just like with any other form of physical training, it's crucial to progress incrementally. Start with simpler exercises and gradually advance to more complex and demanding ones as your strength increases. This not only ensures effectiveness but also minimizes the risk of injury.

Incorporate Variety

While repetition is essential for mastery, monotony can lead to burnout and a lack of interest. A balanced routine that incorporates a range of exercises is the key to staying engaged and challenging your core in multiple ways.

Be Consistent

Consistency is arguably more important than intensity when it comes to core strength development. Aim for shorter, more frequent sessions rather than infrequent, intense workouts. This approach will allow for better muscle recovery and more sustainable progress.

Mind Your Form

Execution trumps everything. Bad form not only reduces the efficacy of the exercise but also increases the risk of injury. Whether you're a beginner or an experienced individual, always prioritize form over speed or the number of repetitions.

Listen to Your Body

While it's natural to feel some level of discomfort when trying new exercises, pain is a red flag. Your body knows its limits, so listen to it. If an exercise causes pain, stop immediately and consult a healthcare provider if needed.

Pair Exercises with Proper Nutrition and Hydration

Muscle growth and recovery are as much about what you eat and drink as they are about how you exercise. A balanced diet rich in protein, healthy fats, and essential vitamins and minerals, coupled with adequate hydration, can significantly enhance your progress.

Assess and Adapt

Lastly, remember that fitness is a dynamic process. What may work today might not be as effective tomorrow. Regular assessments, either through personal observation or with the help of a healthcare provider, can provide valuable insights. Use these assessments to adapt and evolve your core-strengthening routine.

Exercise Guidelines for Seniors

Before we proceed to the exercises, here are some additional guidelines specifically tailored for seniors:

1. **Consult Your Doctor**: Always consult your healthcare provider before starting any new exercise regimen, especially if you have existing health issues or concerns.

2. **Warm-Up**: Always start with a 5-10 minute warm-up. Gentle stretching or walking can prepare your body for more strenuous activity.

3. **Cool Down**: Similar to the warm-up, a cool-down period of light stretching or walking helps your body transition out of the exercise mode, reducing the risk of muscle soreness and injury.

4. **Safety First**: For seniors, safety is paramount. Make sure the exercise area is clear of hazards. Wear appropriate clothing and footwear, and consider exercising with a partner or under supervision, especially in the beginning.

How to Exercise your core

Boosting your core strength isn't just about focusing on abdominal workouts. Your core is actually a complex network of muscles that stretch across your entire torso—from beneath your ribs down to your pelvis and from one side to the other, extending down your back to your glutes. In fact, your core is home to around 35 muscles, both big and small. The key is to diversify your workouts so you're not over-exerting the same muscle groups. When you engage a wide range of these muscles, you lay down a strong foundation that essentially acts as the link between your body's upper and lower halves. This robust core connection enhances the performance of your arms and legs, letting them function at their peak. Now, let's explore some top strategies for enhancing your core strength.

The upcoming chapters will introduce a variety of exercises, broken down by difficulty level, to help you develop a strong core. These will range from fundamental movements that almost anyone can do, to more challenging exercises meant for those who have already built up some core strength. Armed with the foundational knowledge outlined in this chapter, you'll be better equipped to approach these exercises with the proper mindset and techniques for effective and safe strengthening of your core.

SEATED CORE EXERCISES

Ready to have your mind blown? Believe it or not, you can actually supercharge your core without ever leaving your seat! Yup, seated exercises are the unsung heroes of low-impact, safe, and highly effective core conditioning. They're not just game-changers, they're life-changers, especially if you've been sidelined by a stroke, a fall, or any other event that's weakened your core. Practicing seated workouts can help you bounce back with better strength and balance, while also reducing your chances of taking a tumble.

But hold on, there's more! Seated exercises are a godsend for anyone who dreads the thought of lying down on the floor just to stand back up again. So whether you're wheelchair-bound, or simply dealing with balance or stability issues, seated workouts can help you regain your mojo. Not only will they boost your core strength, but they'll also ramp up your confidence and make daily tasks a breeze.

So, what's the game plan? In this oh-so-exciting chapter, we're diving into twelve stellar seated exercises to redefine your core! All you need is a rock-solid, straight-backed chair without arms. And for that extra layer of security, make sure to position your chair near a table or low counter. You can use it for added support if needed.

Seated Forward Roll-Ups

TARGET MUSCLE GROUPS
Rectus Abdominis, Transverse Abdominis

The Seated Forward Roll-Up! This underrated gem is an amazing way to awaken your core and give your spine some love. It's especially ideal if you're a senior, or anyone looking for an effective, low-impact core exercise. So let's get right into it, shall we?

Here's how to perform a seated forward roll-up:

1. Get Positioned: Take a seat in a chair and stretch your legs out in front of you, resting your heels on the ground while pointing your feet towards your face. Reach your arms out ahead of you and make sure to sit up straight—no slouching or leaning back allowed!

2. Take a Deep Breath: Inhale deeply, filling your lungs and expanding your chest.

3. Curl Down: As you exhale, start to curl your chin toward your chest and roll your upper body forward. Imagine peeling your spine away from the back of the chair, one vertebra at a time.

4. Reach Forward: Extend your arms out in front of you as you continue to roll down, aiming to reach towards your toes. Go as far as you comfortably can, but it's totally fine if you can't touch your toes.

5. Hold and Inhale: Pause for a moment at your maximum stretch, take a deep breath in.

6. Roll Back Up: On your exhale, reverse the motion by slowly rolling back up, stacking one vertebra at a time until you're back in the seated upright position.

Seated Bicycle

Seated Bicycle exercise is typically performed while sitting. It is an effective core workout that also engages your lower body.

Here's how:

1. Sit erectly on a workout bench, chair, or box, ensuring your ribcage is aligned over your hips and your feet are positioned flat on the ground, separated at hip-width. Put your hands at the back of your head.

2. As you breathe out, elevate your right leg and rotate your upper body to bring your right knee inward, making contact with your left elbow.

3. Bring your right foot back down to its original position to complete one repetition. Next, elevate your left foot and rotate your upper body to make your right elbow come into contact with your lifted left knee.

4. Keep switching sides and complete 10 repetitions for each side.

Seated Side Bends

The perfect exercise for oblique love and a side of spine mobility. Ideal for everyone, including seniors and those looking for low-impact exercise options, this move adds some much-needed zest to your core routine. Ready to bend it like a pro?

Here's how:

1. The Perfect Seat: Start by sitting tall in a sturdy, armless chair with your feet planted firmly on the floor, hip-width apart.

2. Arm Positioning: Rest your arms down by your sides, palms facing inward.

3. Engage the Core: Take a deep breath and engage your core muscles, as if you're bracing for a tickle attack.

4. The Bend: On an exhale, lean your upper body to one side, sliding one hand down toward the floor while the other hand slides up your side.

5. Pause and Breathe: Hold the side bend for a moment, inhaling deeply.

6. Return to Center: On the exhale, use your core muscles to bring your body back to the upright position.

7. Switch Sides: Now, it's time to give the other side some love. Repeat steps 4-6 for the opposite side.

Remember, make each bend slow and controlled. The aim isn't how far you can bend, but how well you can engage your core muscles while doing it.

Seated Half Roll-Backs

TARGET MUSCLE GROUPS
Rectus Abdominis, Transverse Abdominis

How to Do It:

1. Take a seat in a chair, making sure your knees are bent and your feet are firmly planted on the floor. Raise your arms to chest level, forming a circle in front of you. Maintain a straight back and avoid slumping or reclining in the chair.

2. With your feet firmly planted on the ground and your arms forming a loop in front of your chest, start to curve your back. As you do, envision hollowing out your abdominal muscles like you're scooping them inward.

3. When you've reached your limit and can't roll back any more, activate your core muscles and gradually return to the initial seated position.

Seated Leg Lifts

TARGET MUSCLE GROUPS

Rectus Abdominis, Transverse Abdominis, and Obliques

How to Do It:

1. Grab a seat in a chair and bend your left knee so that your left foot is firmly planted on the floor. Meanwhile, extend your right leg straight out. Sit up tall—no hunching or reclining allowed!

2. Tighten your core and elevate your right leg, aiming to lift it as high as you comfortably can without letting your back sink. Hold that position for a moment, and then gently lower your foot back down to the ground.

Seated Dead Bug

Rectus Abdominis, Transverse Abdominis, and Obliques

Though the name might not be the most appealing, this exercise is fantastic for honing in on both your upper and lower abs.

To execute the "dead bug" move, grab a sturdy chair you can recline in while maintaining a straight back and extended arms. Even a basic folding chair will work well.

How to Do It:

Lean back in the seat until your back is perfectly straight. With your head held high, tighten your core muscles and simultaneously lift your right arm and stretch out your left leg. Maintain this posture for a single second. Go back to the initial stance. Perform the same actions, but this time switch to the opposite arm and leg.

Seated Knee-to-Chest

The Seated Knee-to-Chest exercise is a simple yet effective movement for targeting the lower abdominal muscles and hip flexors. It can also offer some stretching benefits for the lower back and hamstrings. This exercise is often recommended for those who are new to fitness or are looking for a low-impact abdominal exercise. It can also be useful for people with limited mobility or those who prefer to avoid lying down for core exercises.

How to Do It:

1. Sit securely on the chair's edge without feeling as though you're about to tip over.
2. Maintain a straight back while engaging your abdominal and lower back muscles. Puff out your chest.
3. Grasp the sides of the chair with both hands to maintain stability.
4. Extend both legs well ahead of your torso and angle your toes upwards toward the sky. Ensure that your feet are positioned at a diagonal relative to your hips.
5. Gradually lift both legs toward your torso, bending your knees in the process. Aim to bring your knees as near to your chest as you can.

6. Gradually reverse the movement until you return to the initial position, completing one "rep".

You can also choose to perform this motion using just one leg. Just ensure that the other leg is securely positioned on the floor before you start the lift.

Seated Chop

1. Sit upright on a workout bench, chair, or box, aligning your ribcage over your hips, with your feet flat on the ground and spaced hip-width apart.

2. With your hips aligned and your feet fully touching the ground, rotate your upper body to stretch your arms straight out towards the right side of your body.

3. Raise your arms in a slanted direction, crossing them over your torso until they extend past your left shoulder.

4. Return your hands back down across your body to get back to the initial position by moving in the opposite direction.

5. Complete 10 repetitions, then change to the opposite side.

Tummy Twists

This exercise effectively targets the whole core area and also helps in elongating the spine. For optimal abdominal engagement, it's best to use a medicine ball or a comparable item.

1. Pick up a medicine ball or a comparable item.
2. Position yourself on the chair's edge for additional space, ensuring a relaxed but upright posture. Engage your abdominal and lower back muscles to maintain a tight core. Puff your chest outward. Hold the medicine ball in front of you with both hands gripping its sides, keeping your elbows at a bent angle.
3. Raise the ball slightly above your lap and turn your upper torso to the right, ensuring the ball remains in front of you.
4. Turn towards the center, then swivel to the left before finally returning to a central position.
5. Each "rep" corresponds to a complete cycle or rotation.

STANDING EXERCISES

Core exercises that can be done while standing are ideal for seniors looking to engage their core muscles. Each exercise in this category is not only quick and simple but can also be performed in the comfort of your home without requiring any special equipment. Let's delve into each exercisc to understand how it contributes to fortifying your core muscles.

Ticking Clock

The "Ticking Clock" is a standing core exercise that is particularly useful for seniors or those looking to improve their balance, core strength, and stability. It mimics the hands of a clock, requiring you to move your legs in various directions while maintaining an upright posture.

How to Do the Ticking Clock

1. **Start Position**: Stand tall with your feet hip-width apart. Place your hands on your hips or hold them out to the sides for balance. If necessary, stand near a wall or chair for added support.

2. **Engage Core**: Before starting the movement, tighten your core muscles by pulling your belly button towards your spine.

3. **12 O'Clock**: Lift your right leg straight out in front of you as far as comfortably possible. Try to keep the leg straight, engaging your core muscles to maintain balance.

4. **3 O'Clock**: Lower your right leg and then lift it out to the right side, mimicking the 3 o'clock hand on a clock.

5. **6 O'Clock**: Lower your right leg back to the starting position.

6. **9 O'Clock**: Lift your left leg out to the left side, mimicking the 9 o'clock hand on a clock.

7. **12 O'Clock**: Finally, lift your left leg straight out in front of you.

8. **Return**: Bring your left leg back to the starting position.

9. **Reps and Sets**: Complete the full "clock" 3-5 times for each leg. Aim for 2-3 sets.

Tips for Proper Form

- Keep your back straight and posture upright during the entire exercise.

- Make the movements slow and controlled to challenge your core and improve balance.

- If lifting the leg fully is challenging, make smaller lifts. The idea is to engage your core and improve balance.

- As you get more comfortable, try doing the exercise without holding onto a support.

Knee Tuck Extension

The Knee Tuck Extension is a versatile exercise that targets the core muscles, including the abs, obliques, and lower back. This movement also engages your hip flexors and can be beneficial for enhancing balance and stability. Here's how to do the Knee Tuck Extension:

How to Do the Knee Tuck Extension

1. **Start Position**: Stand tall with your feet hip-width apart. Place your hands on your hips or extend them out to the side for added balance. If needed, stand close to a wall or chair for support.

2. **Engage Core**: Tighten your core muscles by pulling your belly button towards your spine. This will help stabilize your lower back and hips during the exercise.

3. **Knee Tuck**: Lift one knee as high as comfortably possible towards your chest. Hold this tuck position for 1-2 seconds.

4. **Leg Extension**: From the tucked position, extend the same leg straight out in front of you. Keep the leg elevated, but you don't have to lift it high; just extending it forward is enough.

5. **Hold**: Maintain the leg extension for another 1-2 seconds, engaging your core to balance.

6. **Return**: Bend the knee back into the tuck position, then lower it down to the starting stance.

7. **Reps and Sets**: Perform 10-12 repetitions on one leg, then switch to the other leg for another 10-12 reps. Aim for 2-3 sets.

Tips for Proper Form

- Keep your back straight and chest lifted throughout the exercise. Avoid leaning backward or forward.

- Make each movement slow and controlled to maximize core engagement.

- If balancing is difficult, you can lightly hold onto a wall or chair for support.

- Always keep your core engaged, pulling your belly button towards your spine for better stability.

Pelvic Tilt

The Pelvic Tilt is a foundational exercise that focuses on strengthening the core muscles, particularly the lower abdominal region and the muscles supporting the lower back. It's especially beneficial for people who experience lower back pain or discomfort, and it can serve as a great warm-up before engaging in more intense workouts. It's also particularly suitable for seniors or those who may be new to exercise.

How to Do a Pelvic Tilt

1. **Start Position**: Stand upright with your feet shoulder-width apart, knees slightly bent. Place your hands on your hips or let them hang by your sides.

2. **Engage Core**: Activate your core muscles by pulling your belly button inward towards your spine. This is crucial for stabilizing your lower back.

3. **Neutral Position**: Find a neutral pelvic position by slightly rocking your pelvis forward and backward. Stop when you find the midpoint where your pelvis feels balanced.

4. **Tilt**: From the neutral position, gently tilt your pelvis forward by arching your lower back slightly. Then, tilt your pelvis backward by tucking your tailbone under and flattening your lower back.

5. **Hold**: In each tilted position, hold for a count of 2-3 seconds, feeling the engagement in your lower abdominals and lower back.

6. **Return**: Return to the neutral position and prepare for the next repetition.

7. **Reps and Sets**: Perform 10-15 repetitions of forward and backward tilts, aiming for 2-3 sets.

Tips for Proper Form

- Keep your upper body relaxed, and let the movement originate from your pelvis and lower back.

- Make sure you are breathing normally throughout the exercise. Inhale in the neutral position, and exhale while tilting.

- The movement should be subtle and controlled. Avoid any jerky or exaggerated tilts.

- Keep your knees soft to avoid putting stress on them or locking them out, which could destabilize you.

Torso Twists

The Torso Twist is an excellent exercise for targeting the oblique muscles and improving core strength. It also helps in enhancing spinal mobility and overall stability. This exercise is often used in warm-up routines or as a part of core-focused workouts. It's also suitable for seniors who are looking to maintain or improve their trunk mobility and core strength.

How to Do Torso Twists

1. **Start Position**: Stand up straight with your feet hip-width apart. Extend your arms out to your sides at shoulder height, or place your hands on your hips for a more controlled movement.

2. **Engage Core**: Before starting, pull your belly button towards your spine to engage your core muscles. This helps in stabilizing the lower back.

3. **Twist**: Rotate your torso to the right as far as comfortably possible, keeping your hips and feet firmly in place. Your head should follow the direction of the torso rotation.

4. **Hold**: Once you reach the maximum point of rotation, hold the position for a count of 1-2 seconds.

5. **Return to Center**: Slowly come back to the starting position.

6. **Twist to the Left**: Repeat the twist on the opposite side.

7. **Reps and Sets**: Complete 10-15 rotations on each side, aiming for 2-3 sets.

Tips for Proper Form

- Keep your hips and lower body stable; the movement should be in the torso only.

- Maintain a slow, controlled motion to fully engage the core muscles.

- Do not rush through the exercise or use momentum to twist, as this may result in strain or injury.

- If standing is difficult, this exercise can also be performed seated.

Wood Chop

The Wood Chop is a dynamic exercise that works multiple muscle groups, including the shoulders, back, and core. This functional movement simulates the action of chopping wood, hence the name. It's particularly effective for building rotational strength and improving stability, making it a suitable addition to any fitness routine, including those designed for seniors.

How to Do the Wood Chop

1. **Start Position**: Stand with your feet hip-width apart. Hold a light dumbbell, medicine ball, or even a water bottle with both hands.

2. **Engage Core**: Pull your belly button toward your spine to activate your core muscles.

3. **Lower Position**: Begin by lowering both arms towards your right hip, keeping your arms straight. As you do this, bend your knees slightly into a mini-squat.

4. **Chop**: In a sweeping diagonal movement, lift the weight from your right hip across your body to above your left shoulder. As you do this, straighten your legs and pivot slightly on your right foot. Your torso should rotate with the movement, but your hips should stay relatively still.

5. **Hold and Return**: At the top of the motion, pause for a moment before reversing the action. Lower the weight back down across your body to your right hip as you bend your knees.

6. **Reps and Sets**: Perform 10-12 repetitions on one side, then switch to the other side for another 10-12 reps. Aim for 2-3 sets.

Tips for Proper Form

- Keep your arms straight but not rigid throughout the exercise to engage your shoulders and core effectively.

- Make sure the movement is smooth and controlled, avoiding any jerky or rushed motions that could result in strain or injury.

- The rotation should come from your torso, not your hips. Your hips should remain facing forward as much as possible throughout the movement.

- To maintain balance, keep your core engaged and your feet firmly planted during the chopping action.

Standing Bicycle Crunch

The Standing Bicycle Crunch is a variation of the traditional bicycle crunch exercise, but it's done in a standing position. This version is more accessible for those who have difficulty getting down onto the floor or prefer to stay on their feet. It targets the core muscles, specifically the obliques, and also involves some coordination and balance. This exercise is suitable for all fitness levels, including seniors.

How to Do the Standing Bicycle Crunch

1. **Start Position**: Stand upright with your feet hip-width apart. Place your hands behind your head with your elbows wide open.

2. **Engage Core**: Activate your core by pulling your belly button in towards your spine. This helps stabilize your lower back during the exercise.

3. **Crunch**: Lift your right knee towards your chest while simultaneously bringing your left elbow down towards the knee.

4. **Hold and Return**: Make contact between your elbow and knee or bring them as close as possible without straining. Hold this position for a brief moment before returning to the starting position.

5. **Alternate**: Now perform the same movement with your left knee and right elbow.

6. **Reps and Sets**: Continue alternating sides for a total of 16-20 reps (8-10 reps per side). Aim for 2-3 sets.

Tips for Proper Form

- Keep your back straight and avoid leaning too far forward or back during the movement. The motion should be focused in the core region.
- Make sure your movements are controlled, not jerky. Rushing through the exercise will reduce its effectiveness and could potentially lead to injury.
- If balance is an issue, you can keep one hand on a chair or against a wall for added support.
- Keep your elbows wide and avoid pulling on your head or neck with your hands.

Diagonal Sit Back

The Diagonal Sit Back is an effective core exercise that targets the obliques, lower back, and even the glutes. It adds a rotational component to the traditional squat or sit-back motion, increasing the engagement of the oblique muscles.

How to Do the Diagonal Sit Back

1. **Start Position**: Begin by standing with your feet about shoulder-width apart. Extend your arms out in front of you at shoulder height.

2. **Engage Core**: Activate your core muscles by pulling your belly button in towards your spine. This will help stabilize your lower back.

3. **Initial Movement**: Begin by bending your knees slightly, as if you're going into a shallow squat.

4. **Diagonal Motion**: As you continue to lower yourself, rotate your upper body and arms diagonally to the right, aiming to sit back and towards the right side.

5. **Depth**: Lower yourself until you feel a good engagement in your obliques, but don't go too far to the point of discomfort or imbalance.

6. **Hold and Return**: Pause for a moment at the bottom of the movement, then push through your feet to return to the starting position.

7. **Alternate Sides**: Repeat the movement, but this time rotate your upper body and arms diagonally to the left.

8. **Reps and Sets**: Continue to alternate sides, aiming for 10-12 reps on each side for a total of 20-24 reps. Complete 2-3 sets.

Tips for Proper Form

- Ensure your back remains straight throughout the exercise to avoid strain or injury.
- Keep your movements controlled and smooth. Avoid any jerky or sudden motions.
- Maintain your feet flat on the ground throughout the exercise.
- If balance is a concern, perform this exercise near a wall or sturdy piece of furniture for support.

Lunging Pull-Down

TARGET MUSCLE GROUPS
Rectus abdominis, Transverse abdominis, Latissimus dorsi, Obliques

The Lunging Pull-Down is an effective compound exercise that works multiple muscle groups simultaneously. Specifically, it targets the lats (latissimus dorsi), shoulders, and back, while also engaging the glutes, hamstrings, and quads through the lunge motion. This exercise can offer benefits in terms of both strength and balance, making it suitable for a wide range of fitness levels, including seniors.

How to Do the Lunging Pull-Down

1. **Start Position**: Stand up straight with your feet hip-width apart. If you have access to a resistance band or cable machine, grasp the handles above your head with both hands. Otherwise, you can hold a towel or even imagine you're holding a bar.

2. **Engage Core**: Activate your core muscles by pulling your belly button in towards your spine, which will stabilize your lower back during the exercise.

3. **Lunge**: Step one foot forward into a lunge, bending both knees at a 90-degree angle. The back knee should hover just above the ground, and the front knee should be aligned with the ankle.

4. **Pull-Down**: As you lower into the lunge, perform a lat pull-down by pulling your arms down towards your sides. Squeeze your shoulder blades together at the bottom of the movement.

5. **Return and Reset**: Push off the front foot to return to the starting position while simultaneously raising your arms back above your head.

6. **Alternate Sides**: Perform the lunge and pull-down on the opposite side.

7. **Reps and Sets**: Aim for 10-12 reps on each side for a total of 20-24 reps. Complete 2-3 sets.

Tips for Proper Form

- Keep your back straight and your chest lifted throughout the exercise.

- Make sure to keep your movements smooth and controlled. Jerky or rapid movements can lead to injury.

- Ensure that your front knee doesn't extend past your toes as you lunge.

- Keep the resistance band, towel, or imaginary bar tight as you pull it down, maximizing the contraction in your lats and shoulders.

MAT CORE EXERCISES

For those who prefer a softer surface or just want to add variety to their core exercise regimen, mat exercises offer a comfortable and effective option. Mat exercises can be particularly good for seniors, as they are often lower-impact and can be done in the safety of your home. Below, we break down mat-based core exercises by skill level—beginner, intermediate, and advanced—so you can find what's most appropriate for you.

Preparation: The Importance of the Mat

Before we get started, let's talk about the mat itself. Choose a mat that provides sufficient cushioning to protect your back yet is firm enough to support your weight. This will make the exercises more comfortable and effective.

Forearm Planks

The forearm plank is a classic core exercise that engages multiple muscle groups, including the abs, lower back, shoulders, and legs. Despite its full-body engagement, it is often considered easier on the wrists and shoulders compared to a high plank, which makes it a great option for various fitness levels.

How to Do a Forearm Plank

1. **Start Position**: Begin by lying face down on the floor or a mat. Place your forearms on the ground, with your elbows directly below your shoulders and your hands flat on the ground.

2. **Foot Position**: Extend your legs straight out behind you, toes tucked under. Your feet should be hip-width apart.

3. **Engage Core**: Tighten your core muscles as if you're pulling your belly button towards your spine.

4. **Lift Up**: Push up onto your forearms and toes, lifting your body off the ground. Your body should form a straight line from your shoulders to your heels. Make

sure your hips aren't sagging or piking up; they should be in line with your shoulders and heels.

5. **Hold**: Keep your body as still as possible, and hold this position for as long as you can maintain good form. Beginners may start with 10-20 seconds, while more advanced individuals may aim for 60 seconds or longer.

6. **Breathing**: Breathe normally while holding the plank position. Don't hold your breath.

7. **Disengage**: To disengage, gently lower your body back to the starting position.

Tips for Proper Form

- Keep your neck neutral by looking at a spot on the floor a few inches in front of your hands.

- Ensure your back is flat, and avoid rounding your shoulders.

- Do not let your hips sag or rise too high.

- Engage your core throughout the exercise.

Modifications and Variations

1. **Knee Plank**: If a full plank is too challenging, you can perform the exercise with your knees on the ground.

2. **Side Forearm Plank**: To target the obliques, transition into a side plank by rotating your body so that you're resting on one forearm with the opposite arm extended towards the sky.

Superman

TARGET MUSCLE GROUPS

Obliques, Lower Back, Erector Spinae, Glutes

The Superman exercise is a bodyweight movement that focuses on strengthening the muscles of the lower back, glutes, and hamstrings. It also engages the upper back and shoulders, making it a great posterior chain exercise.

How to Do the Superman Exercise

1. **Start Position**: Lie face down on the floor or on a mat. Extend your arms straight out in front of you, palms facing down. Your legs should be straight and together.

2. **Engage Core**: Tighten your core muscles as if pulling your belly button towards your spine.

3. **Lift Up**: Lift both your arms and legs off the ground as high as they will go. Your body should resemble the shape of the letter "U" from the side. Try to lift your limbs and chest as high off the ground as possible while keeping your neck neutral. The aim is to put the work into your back muscles, not your neck.

4. **Hold**: Maintain this position for 2-5 seconds, depending on your comfort and strength level.

5. **Lower Down**: Slowly lower your arms, chest, and legs back to the starting position.

6. **Reps**: Perform 10-15 repetitions for 2-3 sets, or as many as you can manage with good form.

Tips for Proper Form

- Keep your head and neck in a neutral position throughout the exercise. Don't look up or down, but rather keep your gaze fixed on the floor.

- Engage your core and glutes throughout the movement to support your lower back.

- Lift your arms and legs simultaneously for balanced muscle engagement.

- Avoid jerky movements; make sure to lift and lower your body in a controlled manner.

Variations

1. **Superman with a Hold**: For added intensity, hold the 'up' position for a longer duration.

2. **Alternating Superman**: Lift the opposite arm and leg simultaneously, rather than lifting both arms and both legs. This works similar muscle groups but allows for more focus on each side.

Glute Bridges

TARGET MUSCLE GROUPS

Glutes, Hamstrings, Lower Back, Rectus Abdominis, Transverse Abdominis

The Glute Bridge is a versatile exercise primarily targeting the glutes, hamstrings, and lower back, while also engaging your core and hip muscles. It's excellent for improving hip mobility and strengthening the posterior chain.

How to Do a Glute Bridge

1. **Start Position**: Lie on your back on a flat surface or exercise mat. Bend your knees and place your feet flat on the floor, hip-width apart. Your arms should be at your sides, palms facing down.

2. **Engage Core**: Before you begin, tighten your core muscles, pulling your belly button towards your spine.

3. **Lift Hips**: Press through your heels and squeeze your glutes to lift your hips off the floor. Your body should form a straight line from your shoulders to your knees at the top of the movement.

4. **Hold**: Pause at the top for 1-3 seconds, making sure your hips are lifted and your glutes are engaged.

5. **Lower Down**: Slowly lower your hips back to the starting position.

6. **Reps and Sets**: Perform 10-15 repetitions for 2-3 sets.

Tips for Proper Form

- Keep your feet flat on the floor and press through your heels as you lift your hips.

- Ensure your knees are in line with your feet and do not cave inward.

- Keep your head and neck in a neutral position. Do not strain your neck by looking up or tucking your chin.

- Make sure you're lifting your hips by engaging your glutes, not your lower back.

Variations and Progressions

1. **Single-Leg Glute Bridge**: For a more challenging variation, extend one leg out straight while performing the bridge. This increases the load on the supporting leg.

2. **Glute Bridge with Resistance Band**: Place a resistance band around your thighs, just above the knees, to add external resistance to the movement.

3. **Glute Bridge Hold**: Instead of performing repetitions, lift your hips and hold the bridge position for an extended period, such as 20-30 seconds or longer.

Dead Bug

The Dead Bug exercise is a popular core-strengthening exercise that targets the abs, obliques, and lower back. It's designed to improve stability, balance, and coordination. The Dead Bug is particularly good for working your core while minimizing the stress on your lower back, making it a safe and effective exercise for people of all fitness levels.

How to Do the Dead Bug Exercise

1. **Start Position**: Lie on your back on a flat surface or exercise mat. Lift your legs so that your knees are bent at a 90-degree angle over your hips. Your arms should be extended straight up towards the ceiling, directly over your shoulders.

2. **Engage Core**: Tighten your core muscles as if pulling your belly button towards your spine. This engagement is crucial for the effectiveness of the exercise and the safety of your lower back.

3. **Extend Limbs**: Slowly lower your right arm and left leg towards the floor while keeping your lower back

pressed into the floor. Your arm and leg should hover just above the ground, without touching it.

4. **Return to Start**: Slowly bring your arm and leg back to the starting position.

5. **Switch Sides**: Repeat the movement with your left arm and right leg.

6. **Reps and Sets**: Perform 10-12 repetitions on each side for 2-3 sets, or as many as you can manage with good form.

Tips for Proper Form

- Keep your lower back flat against the floor throughout the exercise. If you notice an arch forming, reset your position and engage your core more tightly.

- Make sure to move your limbs slowly and deliberately to maximize core engagement and minimize momentum.

- Your limbs should hover just above the ground during each rep; they should not touch the floor.

- Keep your neck and head relaxed on the floor. The work should come from your core, not your neck.

Variations and Progressions

1. **Dead Bug with Resistance**: To make the exercise more challenging, hold a light dumbbell in your hands and/or strap ankle weights to your feet.

2. **Dead Bug with Exercise Ball**: Hold an exercise ball between one arm and the opposite knee to engage your coordination and focus further.

3. **Reverse Dead Bug**: Instead of extending your limbs away from you, start with them extended and then draw your elbow and knee toward each other, crunching your core.

Mountain Climber

The Mountain Climber is a dynamic exercise that works multiple muscle groups, including the core, shoulders, and legs. It's also a great cardio workout that can help improve endurance and agility.

How to Do Mountain Climbers

1. **Start Position**: Begin in a high plank position with your hands directly under your shoulders and your legs fully extended behind you. Your body should form a straight line from your head to your heels.

2. **Engage Core**: Tighten your core muscles, pulling your belly button towards your spine.

3. **Initial Movement**: Bring one knee towards your chest, keeping your toes off the ground. This is your starting position.

4. **Switch Legs**: Explosively switch the position of your legs, extending the bent leg back and bringing the opposite knee towards your chest.

5. **Maintain Position**: Keep your upper body as stable as possible, with your hands remaining in their initial position and your core engaged. Your body should remain in a straight line.

6. **Reps and Sets**: Perform the movement for 30-60 seconds or aim for 15-20 reps on each leg for 2-3 sets.

Tips for Proper Form

- Ensure your hands are positioned directly under your shoulders to engage the chest and shoulders correctly.

- Keep your core engaged throughout the exercise to maintain stability and protect your lower back.

- Maintain a brisk and controlled pace. Too slow, and you lose the cardio benefit; too fast, and you may compromise your form.

- Keep your hips level. Avoid letting them sag or pike up as you perform the movements.

Variations and Progressions

1. **Cross-Body Mountain Climbers**: Bring each knee towards the opposite elbow to engage the obliques more intensely.

2. **Mountain Climbers with Sliders**: Place your feet on sliders or small towels. This makes the exercise more challenging and engages your core even more.

3. **Slow Mountain Climbers**: Perform the exercise slowly to focus more on muscle engagement and less on the cardiovascular aspect.

4. **High Knee Mountain Climbers**: Bring your knee as close to your chest as possible for a deeper range of motion.

Segmental Rotation

The Segmental Rotation exercise is a gentle movement primarily aimed at improving spinal mobility and core stability. It also helps in stretching the lower back and oblique muscles. This is an excellent exercise for individuals who are recovering from back issues, as well as for those looking to add a functional movement into their workout routine.

How to Do Segmental Rotation

1. **Start Position**: Lie on your back on a flat surface or an exercise mat. Bend your knees and place your feet flat on the floor, about hip-width apart. Your arms should be extended out to your sides, palms facing down.

2. **Engage Core**: Tighten your core muscles by pulling your belly button towards your spine. This helps to protect your lower back during the movement.

3. **Initial Rotation**: Slowly drop both knees to one side, trying to bring them as close to the floor as possible without lifting your opposite shoulder off the ground.

4. **Hold**: Hold the position for a couple of seconds, breathing deeply and feeling the stretch along your spine and lower back.

5. **Return to Center**: Slowly bring your knees back to the starting position, engaging your core muscles to do the lifting.

6. **Switch Sides**: Repeat the rotation, dropping your knees to the opposite side this time.

7. **Reps and Sets**: Perform 8-12 repetitions on each side for 2-3 sets.

Tips for Proper Form

- Keep your shoulders flat on the floor throughout the exercise to maximize spinal rotation and stretch.

- Move slowly and in a controlled manner to ensure that you're engaging the correct muscles and to avoid any strain on the lower back.

- Breathe deeply and relax into the stretch, allowing your muscles to naturally lengthen.

Variations and Progressions

1. **Leg Extension**: As you bring your knees back to center, you can extend one leg fully, then return to the bent-knee position before rotating to the other side.

2. **Foot Lift**: For an added challenge, lift the foot of the top leg while in the rotated position, then place it back down before returning to the center.

3. **Arm Reach**: As you rotate your knees to one side, reach your opposite arm towards the ceiling and then back over your head, providing an additional stretch to the upper torso.

Side Plank

The Side Plank is a powerful isometric exercise that targets the obliques, while also engaging the shoulders, back, and hips. This exercise is particularly good for enhancing core strength and stability.

How to Do a Side Plank

1. **Start Position**: Lie on your side with your legs fully extended. Stack your feet on top of each other and place your elbow directly under your shoulder.

2. **Engage Core**: Tighten your core muscles as if you're pulling your belly button towards your spine.

3. **Lift Hips**: Press down through your elbow and feet, lifting your hips and body off the floor. Your body should form a straight line from your head to your heels.

4. **Arm Position**: Your free arm can either be placed on your hip or extended towards the ceiling, depending on your comfort level.

5. **Hold**: Maintain this position for 20-30 seconds, or as long as you can maintain good form.

6. **Lower Down**: Slowly lower your hips back to the starting position.

7. **Switch Sides**: Make sure to perform the exercise on both sides for balanced muscle development.

8. **Reps and Sets**: Aim to hold the side plank for an equal amount of time on each side, and perform 2-3 sets.

Tips for Proper Form

- Make sure your elbow is directly under your shoulder to avoid putting undue stress on the shoulder joint.

- Keep your hips lifted throughout the exercise; avoid letting them sag towards the ground.

- Keep your head in a neutral position, in line with your spine.

- Ensure your body forms a straight line from head to heel. Avoid bending at the hips or rounding the spine.

Variations and Progressions

1. **Side Plank with Leg Lift**: While in the side plank position, lift the top leg towards the ceiling for added difficulty.

2. **Side Plank with Rotation**: From the side plank position, rotate your free arm under your body and then back up to the starting position.

3. **Side Plank Dips**: Lower your hips towards the ground and then lift them back up into the side plank position to engage your obliques more dynamically.

4. **Extended Arm Side Plank**: Instead of resting on your elbow, perform the plank with your arm fully extended and your hand flat on the ground. This increases the difficulty and engages the shoulder more intensely.

Alternating Superhero

TARGET MUSCLE GROUPS

Rectus abdominis, Transverse abdominis, Obliques, Erector spinae

The Alternating Superhero exercise, sometimes also known as the Alternating Superman, is a full-body exercise that primarily targets the muscles in your lower back, glutes, shoulders, and core. It is particularly beneficial for improving posture, balance, and spinal stability.

How to Do Alternating Superhero

1. **Start Position**: Lie flat on your stomach on an exercise mat or flat surface. Extend your arms straight out in front of you, and keep your legs straight, with toes pointing towards the ground.

2. **Engage Core**: Tighten your core muscles, pulling your belly button up towards your spine to protect your lower back.

3. **Initial Lift**: Lift your right arm and left leg off the ground simultaneously. Extend them upwards as far as comfortably possible, while keeping your head in a neutral position.

4. **Hold**: Maintain the lifted position for 2-3 seconds, focusing on engaging the muscles in your lower back, glutes, and shoulders.

5. **Lower Down**: Gently lower your right arm and left leg back to the starting position.

6. **Switch Sides**: Repeat the lift with your left arm and right leg.

7. **Reps and Sets**: Perform 10-15 repetitions for each pair of limbs, aiming for 2-3 sets.

Tips for Proper Form

- Keep your head and neck in a neutral position, in line with your spine. Avoid straining your neck by looking up or tucking your chin to your chest.

- Perform the movements in a slow, controlled manner to maximize muscle engagement.

- Make sure to breathe; inhale on the way up and exhale as you return to the starting position.

- Ensure you're lifting your limbs by engaging your back and glute muscles, rather than relying on momentum.

One-Legged Crunch

TARGET MUSCLE GROUPS
Rectus abdominis, Transverse abdominis

The One-Legged Crunch is an effective abdominal exercise that targets the rectus abdominis, also known as the "six-pack" muscles, while also engaging the obliques and lower back. The exercise provides a balanced core workout and helps improve overall stability and posture.

How to Do a One-Legged Crunch

1. **Start Position**: Lie on your back on a flat surface or an exercise mat. Bend your knees and place your feet flat on the floor, about hip-width apart. Place your hands lightly behind your head or crossed over your chest.

2. **Engage Core**: Activate your core muscles by pulling your belly button towards your spine. This will help stabilize your lower back throughout the exercise.

3. **Leg Position**: Lift one leg off the floor, bending the knee at a 90-degree angle so that the thigh is vertical and the calf is parallel to the ground.

4. **Crunch Movement**: Exhale as you lift your head, shoulders, and upper back off the ground, aiming to

bring your chest towards your lifted knee. Keep your neck relaxed and in line with your spine.

5. **Hold**: Pause at the top of the crunch for a second, engaging your abdominal muscles.

6. **Return**: Inhale as you lower your upper body back to the starting position, but keep the leg lifted.

7. **Reps and Sets**: Perform 10-15 repetitions on one leg, then switch to the other leg for another 10-15 repetitions. Aim for 2-3 sets.

Tips for Proper Form

- Do not pull on your neck or head with your hands. This can cause strain and does not effectively engage the abdominal muscles.

- Keep your lower back pressed into the floor to avoid arching, which can lead to back pain.

- Make sure to breathe properly, exhaling on the way up and inhaling as you return to the starting position.

- Keep the movements controlled and deliberate. Quick, jerky movements can reduce the effectiveness of the exercise and increase the risk of injury.

YOUR DAILY GUIDE

You've acquired a structured plan for enhancing your core strength day by day, and our aspiration is for you to persist even after you've turned the last page of this book. Research suggests it can take from 18 days to more than eight months to establish a new habit. While that may appear extensive, the long-term gains make it a worthwhile endeavor.

Maintaining regularity is crucial when initiating a new habit. While committing 5 or 10 minutes daily to core exercises will lead to cumulative benefits, infrequent efforts won't achieve much. Aim for daily consistency but be alert to the signs of overexertion. A day of rest may be necessary if you encounter unusual pain; remember, soreness is acceptable but pain is not.

If you adhere to your daily regimen consistently, you'll gradually notice your core muscles toughening up. Complement that with a nutritious diet and some cardiovascular activities, and you'll not only look better but also reduce your susceptibility to health issues and accidental injuries like falling.

To make this a lifelong habit, willpower isn't the only resource you can draw upon. Here are some practical tips:

Define Your Purpose. List your objectives for focusing on core strength and put that list in a place where you'll regularly see it. Constantly seeing your goals will make your daily regimen feel more like a choice than an obligation.

Use Reminders. If you have access to a smartphone, you can easily program daily alerts to keep you on track. Various apps are available to send you scheduled notifications, or you can use your device's built-in alarm features. If you're more of a traditionalist, sticky notes are an effective way to remind yourself, along with carrying motivational messages like "I'm capable" or "Health is my choice."

Incorporate Enjoyment. To make your daily sessions more engaging, mesh them with activities you take pleasure in— be it your favorite TV series, a lively playlist, or even a cherished call with family members.

Get a Companion. Encourage a friend to join your daily core-strengthening routine and keep each other accountable. Modern technology like video calls ensures that distance is no barrier to your partnership.

In conclusion, we urge you to embark on this journey of crafting a healthier and stronger version of yourself. We salute your proactive steps towards improved mobility and a life less burdened by pain, and wish you ongoing success in your personal growth.